WALL PILATES FOR SENIORS

The Ultimate Guide with 30+ Workouts to Improve Your Strength, Flexibility, and Balance Without Ever Leaving the Ground

SKYLAR TAYLOR

TABLE OF CONTENTS

INTRODUCTION

Dear Beloved Reader,

In the quiet living room of a cozy retirement community, Emma sat with a copy of "Wall Pilates for Seniors." The book had become her trusted companion, guiding her through a transformative journey. At seventy-eight, Emma had initially struggled with balance and stiffness, but the exercises within its pages had become her salvation.

Every day, she followed the simple instructions, pressing her body against the wall, finding newfound strength and flexibility. With each gentle movement, she shed years of physical limitations. Emma's energy surged, her posture improved, and the aches that once plagued her vanished.

But the book offered more than just physical benefits. It gave her a renewed sense of confidence and independence. She could now keep up with her grandchildren and enjoy life to the fullest.

"Wall Pilates for Seniors" had become Emma's fountain of youth, a testament to the incredible resilience of the human spirit.

EXCERSICES

General Guidelines and Tips for Wall Pilates for Seniors

1. Start slowly and gradually increase the intensity and duration of your workouts. Wall Pilates is a low-impact exercise, but it's important to start slowly and listen to your body. Don't push yourself too hard, especially when you're first starting out.

2. Focus on proper form. It's important to do the exercises correctly to avoid injury. If you're not sure how to do an exercise, ask a qualified Pilates instructor for help.

3. Breathe deeply and evenly. Pilates is a mind-body exercise, so it's important to focus on your breath. Breathe deeply and evenly throughout each exercise.

4. Engage your core. Your core muscles are the foundation of your body, so it's important to engage them during every exercise. This will help you maintain proper form and protect your back.

5. Be mindful of your alignment. Make sure your spine is in a neutral position and your shoulders are relaxed.

6. Don't bounce. Pilates exercises are slow and controlled. Don't bounce or jerk your body through the movements.

7. Modify exercises as needed. If an exercise is too difficult, modify it to make it easier. You can also use props, such as a foam roller or resistance band, to help you with certain exercises.

8. Warm up before you start your workout and cool down afterwards. A good warm-up will help to prepare your body for exercise and reduce your risk of injury. A cool-down will help your body to recover from exercise.

9. Drink plenty of water before, during, and after your workout.

10. Listen to your body and take breaks when needed. If you feel any pain, stop the exercise and rest.

Here are some additional tips for seniors:

- Be aware of your balance and avoid exercises that make you feel unstable.

- If you have any joint pain, modify exercises to avoid putting stress on the affected joints.

- If you have any health concerns, talk to your doctor before starting a new exercise program.

Wall Pilates is a great way for seniors to improve their strength, flexibility, and balance. It's a low-impact exercise that can be modified to fit any fitness level. Be sure to follow the general guidelines and tips above to stay safe and get the most out of your workouts.

Exercise One: Wall Push-Ups

- **Introduction:** Wall push-ups are a modified version of traditional push-ups that are easier on the joints. This exercise helps to strengthen the chest, triceps, and shoulders.

- **<u>Instructions:</u>**

  1. Stand facing a wall with your feet shoulder-width apart.

  2. Place your hands on the wall at shoulder height, slightly wider than your shoulders.

  3. Lean forward until your body forms a straight line from your head to your heels.

  4. Bend your elbows and lower your body towards the wall until your chest touches the wall.

  5. Push back up to the starting position.

- Illustration:

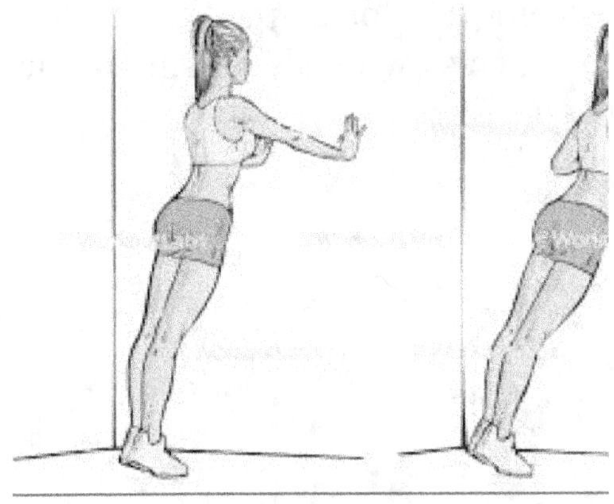

Wall Pushup

- **Sets and Repetitions:** Two sets of Ten to Twelve repetitions

Exercise Two: Wall Squats

- **Introduction:** Wall squats are a great way to strengthen the quadriceps, hamstrings, and glutes. This exercise is also good for improving balance and coordination.

- **Instructions:**

    1. Stand facing a wall with your feet shoulder-width apart.

    2. Lean back against the wall until your back is flat against the wall.

    3. Slide down the wall until your thighs are parallel to the ground, making sure your knees are aligned over your ankles.

4. Hold the position for 10-15 seconds, then slowly slide back up to the starting position.

- Illustration:

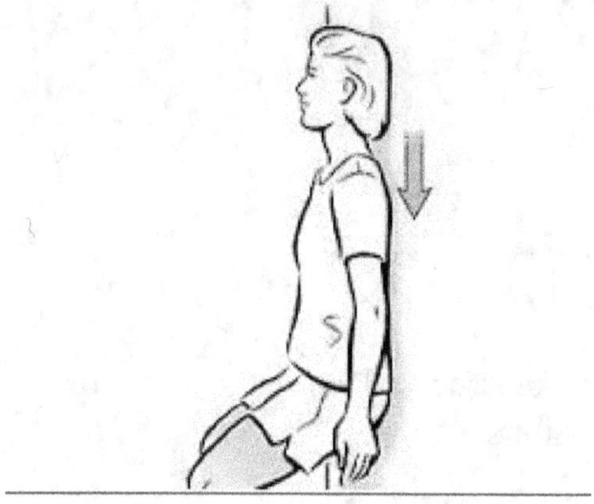

Wall Squats

- **Sets and Repetitions:** Two sets of Ten to Twelve repetitions

Exercise 3: Wall Leg Raises

- **Introduction:** Wall leg raises are a great way to strengthen the hamstrings and glutes. This exercise is also good for improving flexibility and range of motion in the hips.

- **Instructions:**

  1. Lie on your back on the floor with your feet against the wall.

  2. Raise one leg up the wall until it is straight.

  3. Hold the position for 10-15 seconds, then slowly lower your leg back down to the starting position.

  4. Repeat with the other leg.

- Illustration:

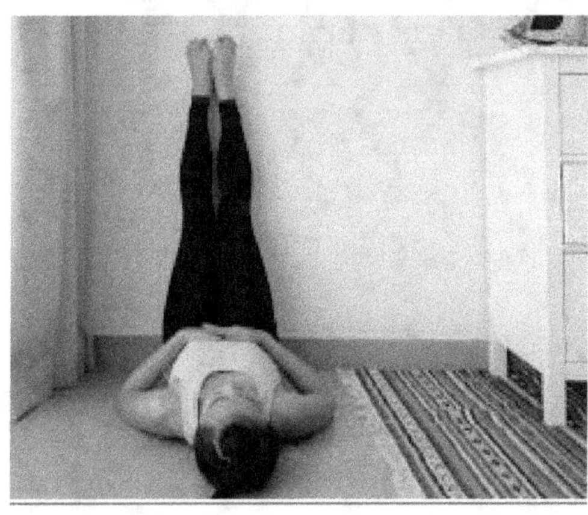

Wall Leg Raises

- **Sets and Repetitions:** Two sets of Ten to twelve repetitions per leg

Exercise 4: Wall Bridge

- **Introduction:** The wall bridge is a great way to strengthen the core muscles, including the abdominals, back, and glutes. This exercise is also good for improving balance and stability.

- **<u>Instructions:</u>**

  1. Lie on your back on the floor with your feet against the wall and your knees bent.

  2. Raise your hips off the floor until your body forms a straight line from your shoulders to your knees.

  3. Hold the position for 10-15 seconds, then slowly lower your hips back down to the starting position.

- Illustration:

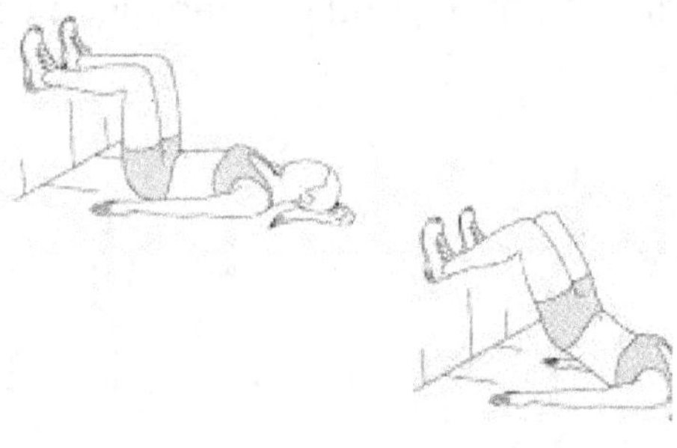

Wall Bridge

- **Sets and Repetitions:** 2 sets of 10-12 repetitions

Exercise 5: *Wall Plank*

- **Introduction:** The wall plank is a great way to strengthen the core muscles, including the abdominals, back, and glutes. This exercise is also good for improving balance and stability.

- **Instructions:**

    1. Start in a push-up position with your forearms on the ground and your hands interlocked.

    2. Place your feet against the wall and walk your feet forward until your body forms a straight line from your head to your heels.

3. Hold the position for as long as you can, maintaining good core engagement.

- Illustration:

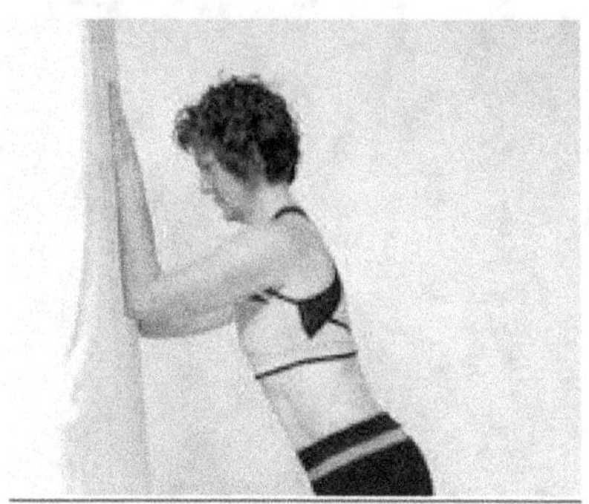

Wall Plank

- **Sets and Repetitions:** 1-2 sets of 30-60 seconds

Exercise 6: Wall Roll-Downs

- **Introduction:** Wall roll-downs are a great way to stretch the spine and hamstrings. This exercise can also help to improve flexibility and range of motion in the back and hips.

- **Instructions:**

  1. Stand facing a wall with your feet shoulder-width apart.

  2. Reach your arms overhead and place your palms on the wall, slightly wider than your shoulders.

3. Slowly roll down the wall, one vertebra at a time, until your fingertips reach the floor.

4. Pause at the bottom for 10-15 seconds, then slowly roll back up the wall to the starting position.

Illustration:

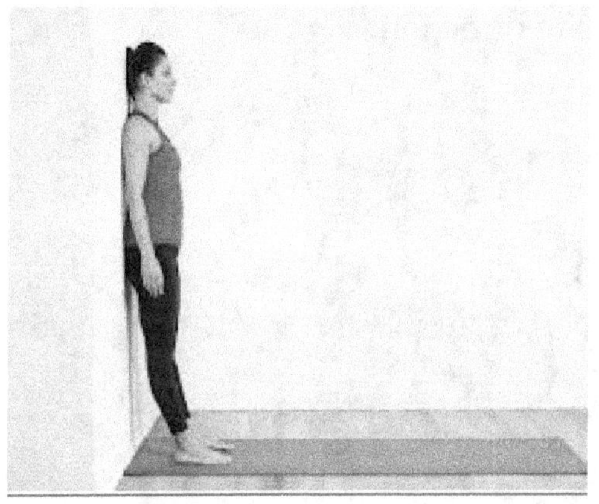

Wall Rolldown

- **Sets and Repetitions:** 1-2 sets of 10-12 repetitions

Exercise 7: Wall Hip Circles

- **Introduction:** Wall hip circles are a great way to warm up the hips and improve flexibility and range of motion. This exercise is also good for strengthening the core muscles.

- **Instructions:**

1. Stand facing a wall with your feet shoulder-width apart.

2. Place your hands on the wall at shoulder height.

3. Slowly make small circles with your hips, moving in a clockwise direction.

4. Do 10-15 circles, then repeat in the opposite direction.

Illustration:

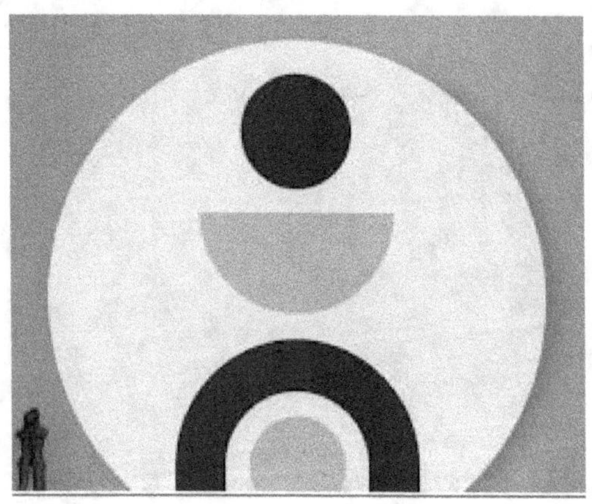

Wall Hip Circles

- **Sets and Repetitions:** Two sets of Ten to Fifteen circles per direction

Exercise 8: Wall Side Plank

- **Introduction:** The wall side plank is a great way to strengthen the core muscles, including the abdominals, obliques, and glutes. This exercise is also good for improving balance and stability.

- **<u>Instructions:</u>**

    1. Start in a push-up position with your right forearm on the ground and your left hand on the wall at shoulder height.

    2. Stack your feet on top of each other and rotate your body so that you are facing the wall.

    3. Raise your hips off the ground until your body forms a straight line from your head to your heels.

    4. Hold the position for as long as you can, maintaining good core engagement.

    5. Repeat on the other side.

Illustration:

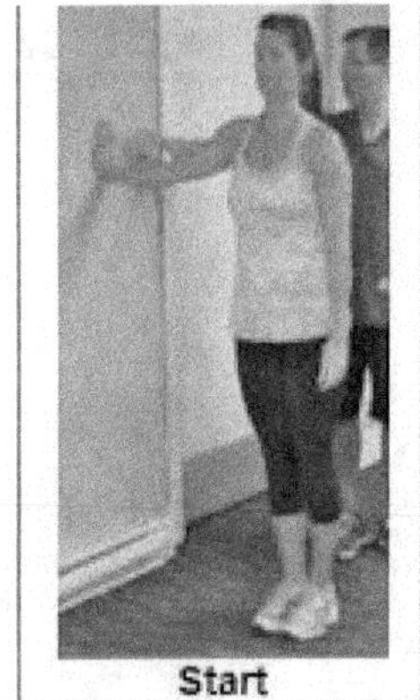

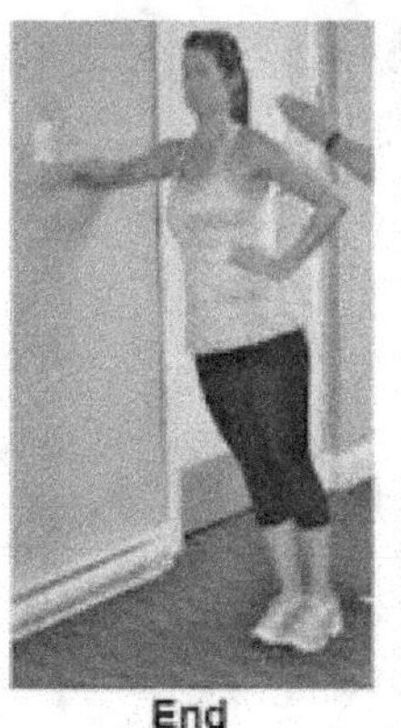

Wall Side Plank

- **Sets and Repetitions:** One to two sets of Thirty-Sixty seconds per side

Exercise 9: Wall Leg Swings

- **Introduction:** Wall leg swings are a great way to warm up the legs and improve flexibility and range of motion in the hips. This exercise is also good for strengthening the hamstrings and glutes.

- **Instructions:**

    1. Stand facing a wall with your feet shoulder-width apart.

    2. Place your hands on the wall at shoulder height.

    3. Swing your right leg forward and back, keeping your leg straight.

    4. Do 10-15 swings, then repeat with the other leg.

Illustration:

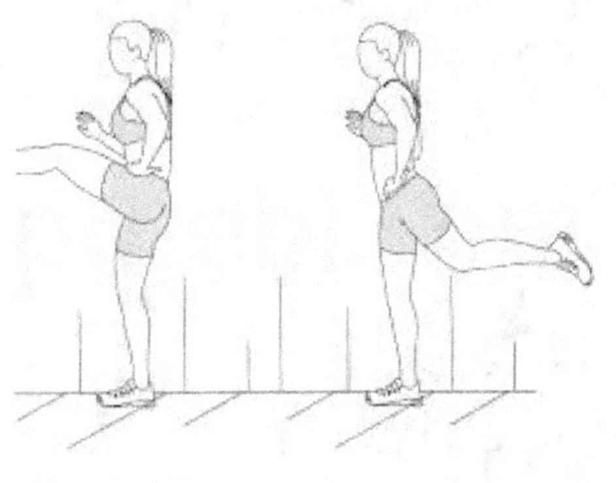

Wall Leg Swings

- **Sets and Repetitions:** Two sets of Ten to Fifteen swings per leg

Exercise 10: Wall Arm Circles

- **Introduction:** Wall arm circles are a great way to warm up the shoulders and improve flexibility and range of motion in the arms and shoulders. This exercise is also good for strengthening the rotator cuff muscles.

- **Instructions:**

    1. Stand facing a wall with your feet shoulder-width apart.

    2. Place your hands on the wall at shoulder height.

    3. Make small circles with your arms in a clockwise direction.

4. Do 10-15 circles, then repeat in the opposite direction.

Illustration:

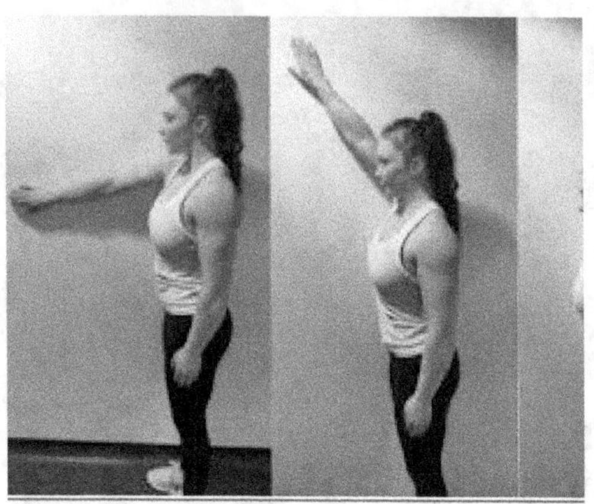

Wall Arm Circles

- **Sets and Repetitions:** Two sets of Ten to Fifteen circles per direction

Exercise 11: *Wall Walk-Ups*

- **Introduction:** Wall walk-ups are a great way to strengthen the hamstrings, glutes, and calves. This exercise is also good for improving balance and coordination.

- **Instructions:**

  1. Stand facing a wall with your feet shoulder-width apart.

  2. Place your hands on the wall at shoulder height.

  3. Walk your feet up the wall until you are in a squatting position, with your knees bent and your thighs parallel to the ground.

  4. Walk your feet back down the wall to the starting position.

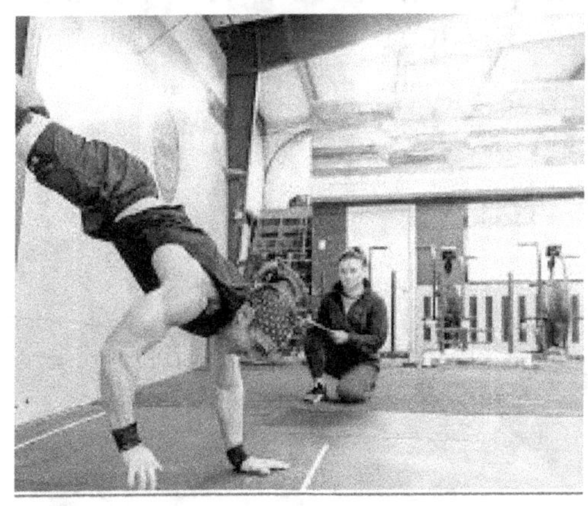

Wall Walkups

- **Sets and Repetitions:** Two sets of Ten to Twelve repetitions

Exercise 12: Wall Bird Dog

- **Introduction:** The wall bird dog is a great way to strengthen the core muscles and improve balance and stability. This exercise is also good for stretching the hamstrings and lower back.

- **Instructions:**

  1. Start on your hands and knees, facing a wall.

  2. Place your hands on the wall at shoulder height, slightly wider than your shoulders.

  3. Extend your right arm and left leg out straight.

  4. Hold the position for 10-15 seconds, then return to the starting position.

  5. Repeat on the other side.

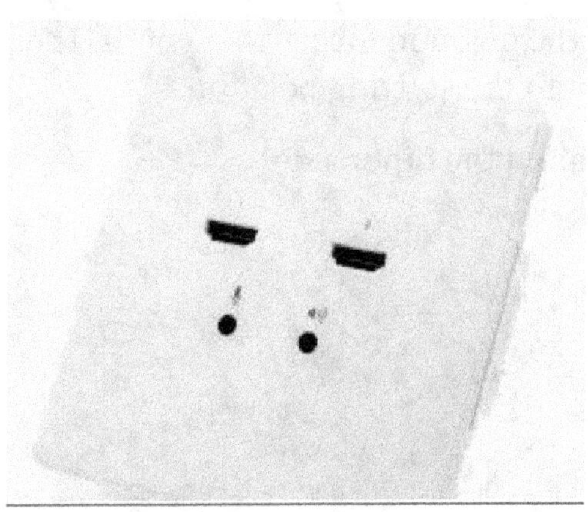

Wall Bird Dog

- **Sets and Repetitions:** Two sets of Ten to Twelve repetitions per side

Exercise 13: Wall Scorpion

- **Introduction:** The wall scorpion is a great way to stretch the spine and hamstrings. This exercise is also good for improving flexibility and range of motion in the back and hips.

- **Instructions:**

  1. Stand facing a wall with your feet shoulder-width apart.

  2. Bend your right leg and place your right foot on the wall, at hip height.

  3. Reach your left arm down and towards your right foot.

4. Hold the position for 10-15 seconds, then return to the starting position.

5. Repeat on the other side.

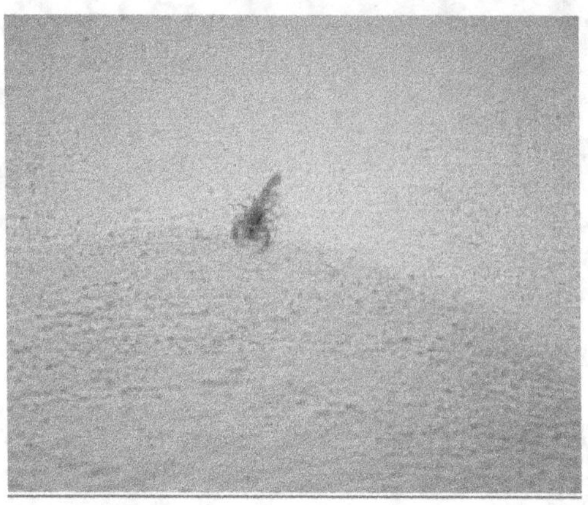

Wall Scorpion

- **Sets and Repetitions:** Two sets of Ten to Twelve repetitions per side

Exercise 14: Wall Chest Opener

- **Introduction:** The wall chest opener is a great way to stretch the chest and shoulders. This exercise is also good for improving flexibility and range of motion in the upper body.

- **Instructions:**

1. Stand facing a wall with your arms outstretched at shoulder height.

2. Place your palms on the wall and lean forward until your chest touches the wall.

3. Hold the position for 10-15 seconds, then slowly return to the starting position.

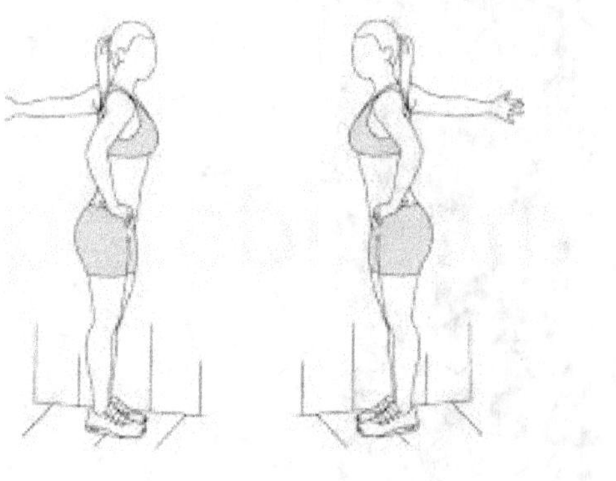

Wall Chest Opener

- **Sets and Repetitions:** Two sets of Ten to Twelve repetitions

Exercise 15: Wall Calf Stretches

- **Introduction:** Wall calf stretches are a great way to stretch the calf muscles. This exercise is also good for improving flexibility and range of motion in the ankles and feet.

- **Instructions:**

    1. Stand facing a wall with your hands on the wall at shoulder height.

    2. Step back with your right leg until you feel a stretch in the back of your right calf.

3. Hold the stretch for 10-15 seconds, then repeat with the other leg.

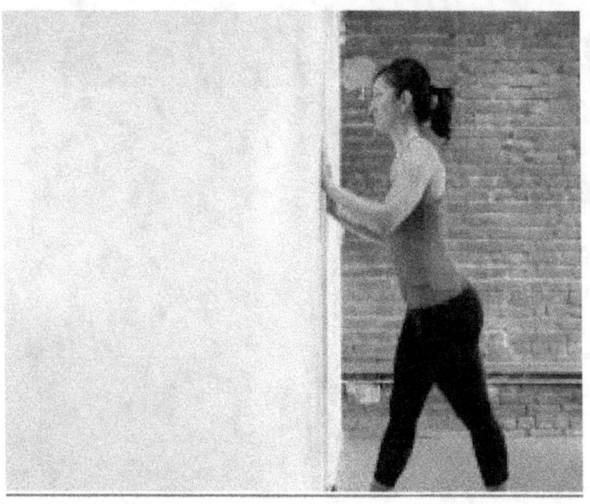

Wall Calf Stretches

- **Sets and Repetitions:** Two sets of Ten to Twelve repetitions per leg

Exercise 16: *Wall Knee Lifts*

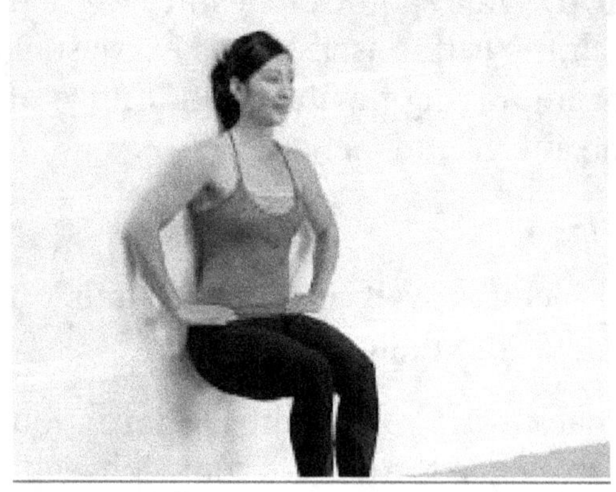

Wall Knee Lifts

- **Introduction:** Wall knee lifts are a great way to warm up the legs and improve flexibility and range of motion in the hips and knees. This exercise is also good for strengthening the hamstrings and quadriceps.

- **Instructions:**

  1. Stand facing a wall with your feet shoulder-width apart.

  2. Place your hands on the wall at shoulder height.

  3. Lift your right knee up towards your chest, keeping your leg straight.

  4. Hold the position for 1-2 seconds, then slowly lower your leg back down to the starting position.

  5. Repeat with the other leg.

- **Sets and Repetitions:** 2 sets of 10-12 repetitions per leg

Exercise 17: Wall Hamstring Stretches

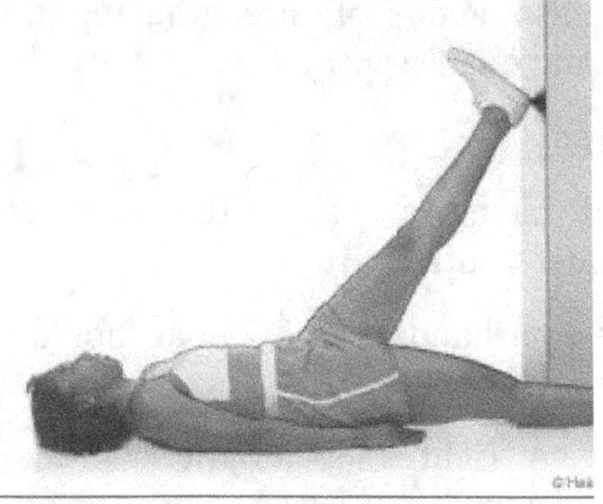

Wall Hamstring Stretches

- **Introduction:** Wall hamstring stretches are a great way to stretch the hamstring muscles. This exercise is also good for improving flexibility and range of motion in the back of the legs.

- **Instructions:**

  1. Stand facing a wall with your feet shoulder-width apart.

  2. Place your right foot on the wall, at knee height.

  3. Keep your right leg straight and lean forward until you feel a stretch in the back of your right hamstring.

4. Hold the stretch for 10-15 seconds, then repeat with the other leg.

- **Sets and Repetitions:** Two sets of Ten to Twelve repetitions per leg

Exercise 18: Wall Ankle Circles

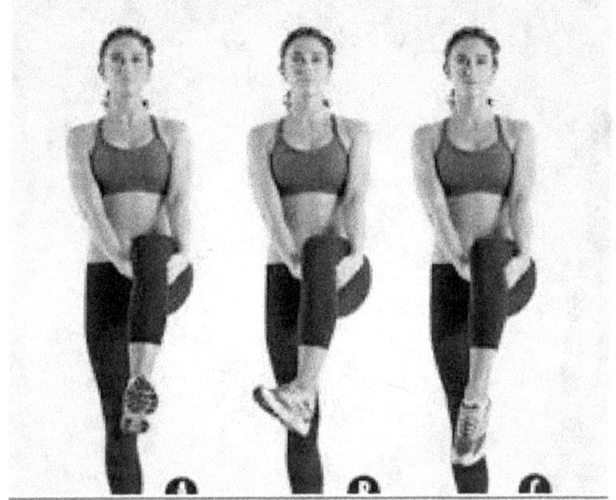

Wall Ankle Circles

- **Introduction:** Wall ankle circles are a great way to warm up the ankles and improve flexibility and range of motion in the ankles and feet. This exercise is also good for strengthening the muscles around the ankles.

- **Instructions:**

    1. Stand facing a wall with your hands on the wall at shoulder height.

    2. Make small circles with your right ankle, in a clockwise direction.

3. Do 10-15 circles, then repeat in the opposite direction.

4. Repeat with the other leg.

- **Sets and Repetitions:** : Two sets of Ten to fifteen circles per leg

Exercise 19: Wall Foot Flexes

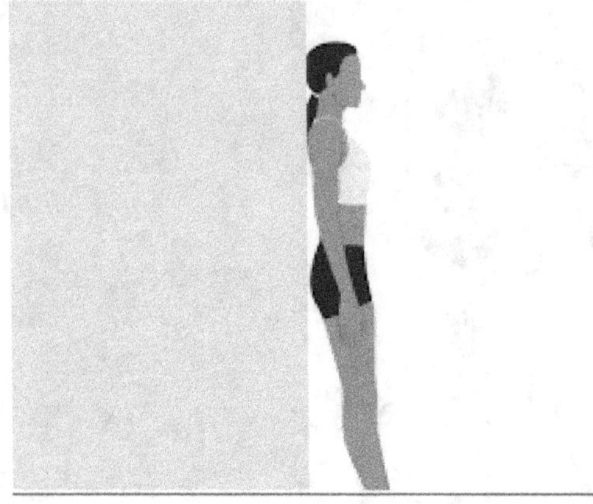

Wall Foot Flexes

- **Introduction:** Wall foot flexes are a great way to warm up the feet and improve flexibility and range of motion in the ankles and feet. This exercise is also good for strengthening the muscles in the feet.

- **Instructions**:

  1. Stand facing a wall with your hands on the wall at shoulder height.

2. Flex your right foot, pointing your toes towards your shin.

3. Hold the position for 1-2 seconds, then slowly relax your foot.

4. Repeat with the other foot.

- **Sets and Repetitions:** Two sets of Ten to twelve repetitions per foot

Exercise 20: Wall Toe Raises

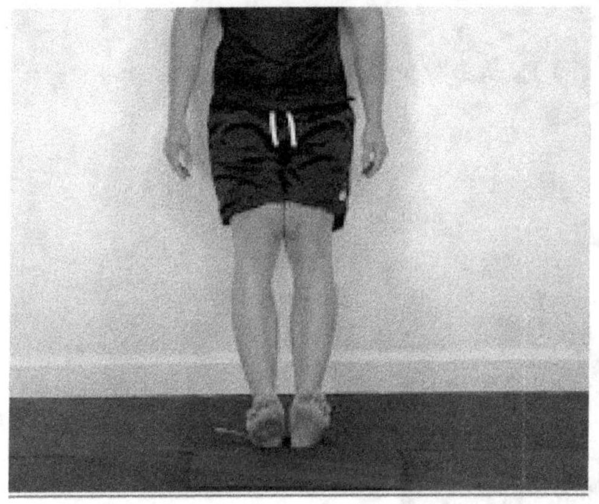

Wall Toe Raises

- **Introduction:** Wall toe raises are a great way to strengthen the calf muscles. This exercise is also good for improving balance and coordination.

- **Instructions:**

    1. Stand facing a wall with your feet shoulder-width apart.

2. Place your hands on the wall at shoulder height.

3. Raise your heels off the ground until you are standing on your toes.

4. Hold the position for 1-2 seconds, then slowly lower your heels back down to the starting position.

- **Sets and Repetitions:** Two sets of Ten to Twelve repetitions

Exercise 21: Wall Leg Slides

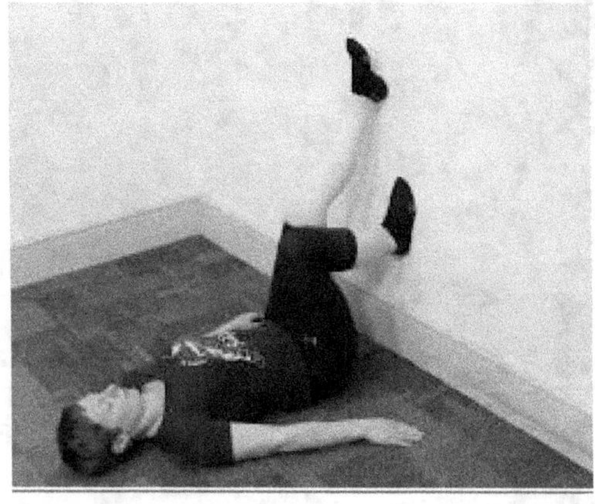

Wall Leg Slides

- **Introduction:** Wall leg slides are a great way to strengthen the hamstrings and glutes. This exercise is also good for improving flexibility and range of motion in the back of the legs.

- **Instructions:**

1. Lie on your back on the floor with your feet against the wall and your knees bent.

2. Slide your right leg up the wall until your leg is straight.

3. Hold the position for 1-2 seconds, then slowly slide your leg back down to the starting position.

4. Repeat with the other leg.

Sets and Repetitions: Two sets of Ten to twelve repetitions per leg

Exercise 22: *Wall Hip Bridges*

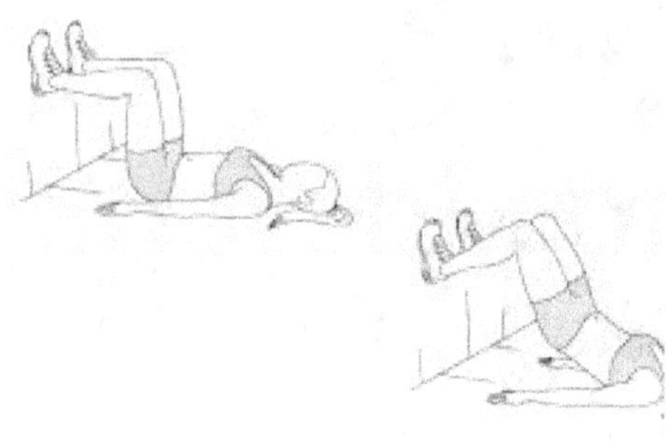

Wall Hip Bridges

- **Introduction:** Wall hip bridges are a great way to strengthen the core muscles, including the abdominals, back, and glutes. This exercise is also good for improving balance and stability.

- **<u>Instructions:</u>**

    1. Lie on your back on the floor with your feet against the wall and your knees bent.

    2. Raise your hips off the ground until your body forms a straight line from your shoulders to your knees.

    3. Hold the position for 1-2 seconds, then slowly lower your hips back down to the starting position.

Sets and Repetitions: Two sets of Ten - Twelve repetitions

Exercise 23: Wall Shoulder Rolls

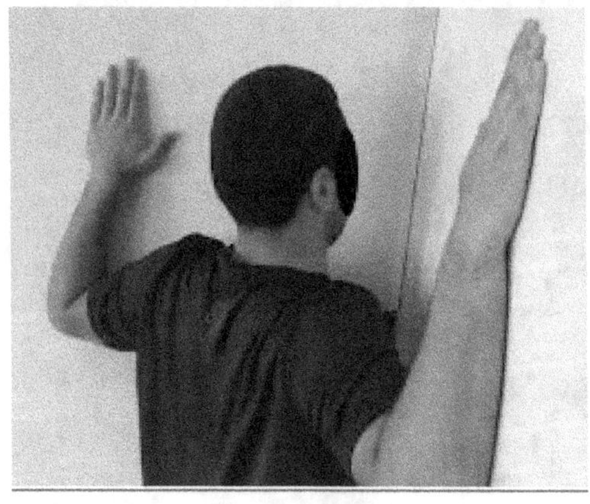

Wall Shoulder Rolls

- **Introduction:** Wall shoulder rolls are a great way to warm up the shoulders and improve flexibility and range of motion in the shoulders and upper back. This exercise is also good for strengthening the rotator cuff muscles.

- **<u>Instructions:</u>**

    1. Stand facing a wall with your feet shoulder-width apart.

    2. Place your hands on the wall at shoulder height, slightly wider than your shoulders.

    3. Make small circles with your shoulders in a clockwise direction.

    4. Do 10-15 circles, then repeat in the opposite direction.

Sets and Repetitions: Two sets of Ten to Fifteen circles per direction

Exercise 24: Wall Chest Stretch

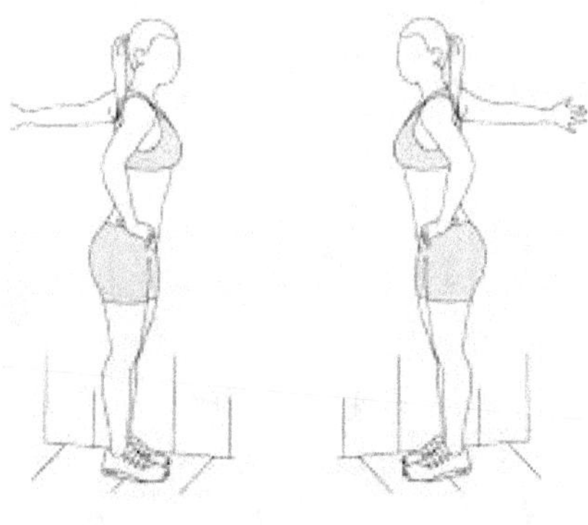

Wall Chest Stretch

- **Introduction:** The wall chest stretch is a great way to stretch the chest and shoulders. This exercise is also good for improving flexibility and range of motion in the upper body.

- <u>**Instructions:**</u>

  1. Stand facing a wall with your arms outstretched at shoulder height.

  2. Place your palms on the wall and lean forward until you feel a stretch in your chest.

  3. Hold the stretch for 10-15 seconds, then slowly return to the starting position.

Sets and Repetitions: Two sets of Ten to Twelve repetitions

Exercise 25: Wall Triceps Stretches

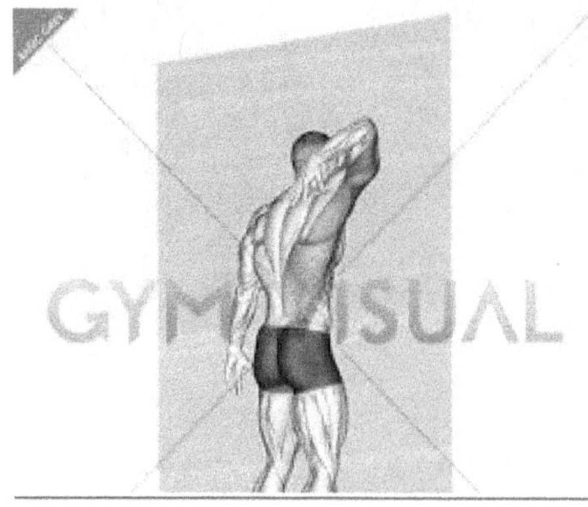

Wall Triceps Stretches

- **Introduction:** Wall triceps stretches are a great way to stretch the triceps muscles. This exercise is also good for improving flexibility and range of motion in the back of the arms.

- <u>**Instructions:**</u>

  1. Stand facing a wall with your feet shoulder-width apart.

  2. Place your right hand on the wall, at shoulder height.

  3. Turn your right hand so that your palm is facing away from the wall.

  4. Step back with your right foot until you feel a stretch in the back of your right triceps.

  5. Hold the stretch for 10-15 seconds, then repeat with the other arm.

Sets and Repetitions: Two sets of Ten – Twelve repetitions per arm

Exercise 26: Wall Heel Slides

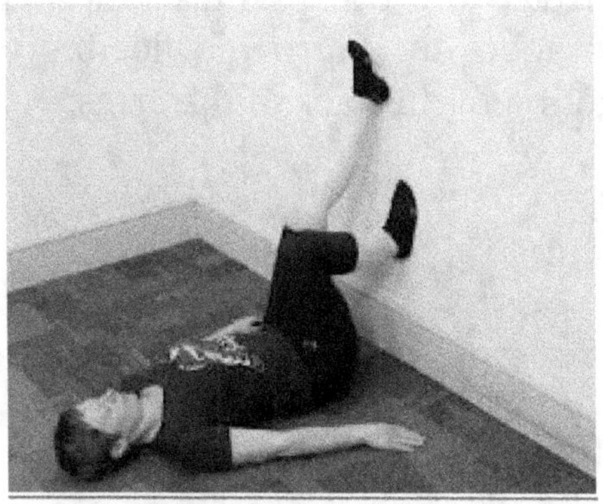

Wall Heel Slides

- **Introduction:** Wall heel slides are a great way to warm up the hamstrings and glutes. This exercise is also good for improving flexibility and range of motion in the back of the legs.

- **Instructions:**

  1. Stand facing a wall with your feet shoulder-width apart.

  2. Place your hands on the wall at shoulder height.

  3. Slide your right heel back towards the wall, keeping your leg straight.

  4. Hold the position for 1-2 seconds, then slowly slide your heel back down to the starting position.

  5. Repeat with the other leg.

Sets and Repetitions: Two sets of ten to Twelve repetitions per leg

Exercise 27: Wall Knee Bends

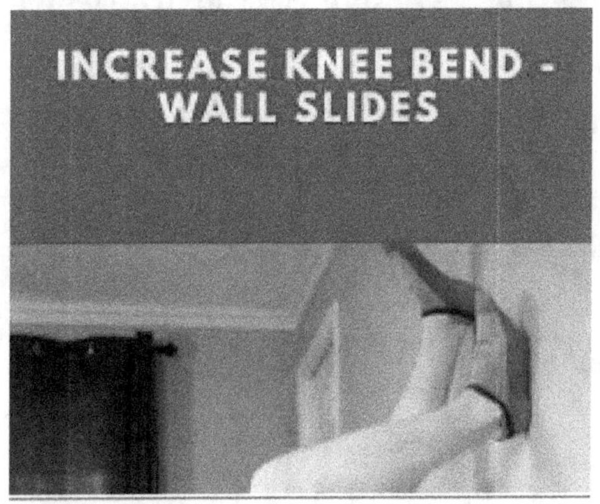

Wall Knee Bends

- **Introduction:** Wall knee bends are a great way to strengthen the quadriceps and hamstrings. This exercise is also good for improving balance and stability.

- **Instructions:**

    1. Stand facing a wall with your feet shoulder-width apart.

    2. Place your hands on the wall at shoulder height.

    3. Bend your knees and lower your body down until your thighs are parallel to the ground.

4. Hold the position for 1-2 seconds, then slowly push back up to the starting position.

Sets and Repetitions: Two sets of Ten to Twelve repetitions

Exercise 28: Wall Calf Raises

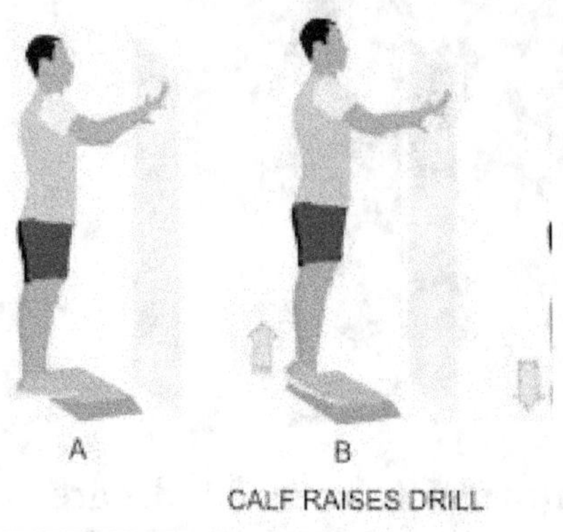

Wall Calf Raises

- **Introduction:** Wall calf raises are a great way to strengthen the calf muscles. This exercise is also good for improving balance and coordination.

- **Instructions:**

    1. Stand facing a wall with your feet shoulder-width apart.

    2. Place your hands on the wall at shoulder height.

3. Raise your heels off the ground until you are standing on your toes.

4. Hold the position for 1-2 seconds, then slowly lower your heels back down to the starting position.

Sets and Repetitions: Two sets of Ten to Twelve repetitions

Exercise 29: Wall Leg Holds

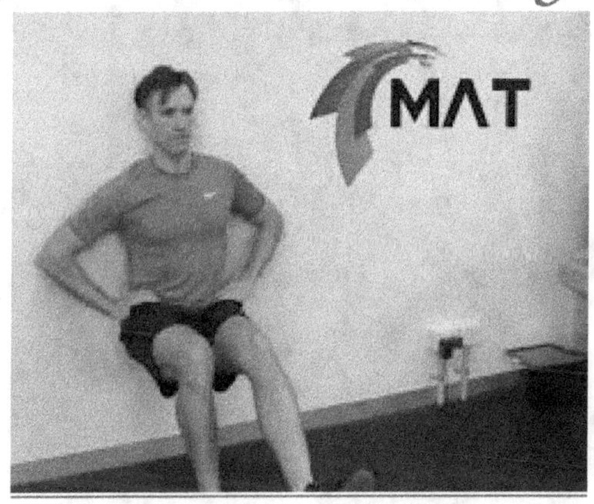

Wall Leg Holds

- Introduction: Wall leg holds are a great way to strengthen the hamstrings and glutes. This exercise is also good for improving balance and stability.

- **Instructions:**

    1. Stand facing a wall with your feet shoulder-width apart.

2. Place your hands on the wall at shoulder height.

3. Lift your right leg off the ground and extend it straight out in front of you.

4. Hold the position for 10-15 seconds, then slowly lower your leg back down to the starting position.

5. Repeat with the other leg.

Sets and Repetitions: : Two sets of Ten to Twelve repetitions per leg

Exercise 30: Wall Arm Circles

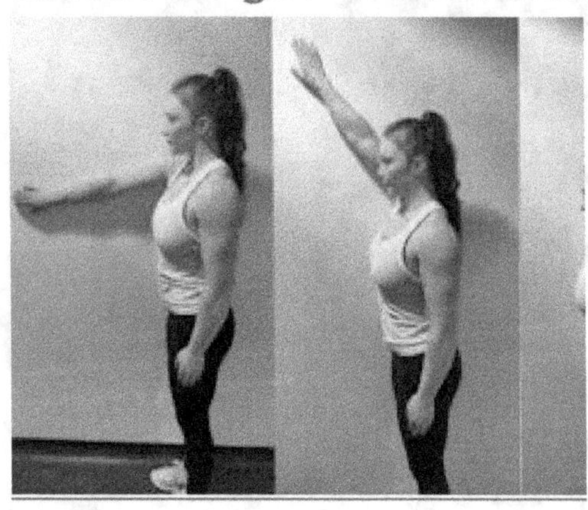

Wall Arm Circles

- **Introduction:** Wall arm circles are a great way to warm up the shoulders and improve flexibility and range of motion in the shoulders and upper back. This exercise is also good for strengthening the rotator cuff muscles.

- **<u>Instructions:</u>**

    1. Stand facing a wall with your feet shoulder-width apart.

    2. Place your hands on the wall at shoulder height, slightly wider than your shoulders.

    3. Make small circles with your arms in a clockwise direction.

    4. Do 10-15 circles, then repeat in the opposite direction.

Sets and Repetitions: Two sets of Ten to fifteen circles per direction.

Motivational Quotes

1. "Pilates is a way to life, not just an exercise program." - Joseph Pilates

2. "Age is just a number. It's never too late to start Pilates." - Unknown

3. "Pilates is a great way to stay strong, flexible, and balanced as you age." - Unknown

4. "Pilates is a low-impact exercise, so it's easy on your joints." - Unknown

5. "Pilates can help improve your posture, reduce pain, and boost your energy levels." - Unknown

6. "Pilates is a mind-body exercise, so it's good for both your physical and mental health." - Unknown

7. "Pilates is a fun and challenging workout that can be modified to fit any fitness level." - Unknown

8. "Pilates is a great way to connect with other seniors and build a supportive community." - Unknown

9. "Pilates can help you age gracefully and live your best life." - Unknown

10. "Pilates is the secret to a healthy and happy life." - Unknown

11. "You're never too old to start Pilates." - Unknown

12. "Pilates is the perfect way to stay fit and healthy as you age." - Unknown

13. "Pilates is a gift you can give yourself." - Unknown

14. "Pilates is the best way to invest in your future." - Unknown

15. "Pilates is the key to a lifetime of health and happiness." - Unknown

I hope these quotes motivate you to start or continue your Pilates practice!

CONCLUSION

Thank you from the depths of our hearts for choosing "Wall Pilates for Seniors" as your guide to improved health and well-being. Your decision to embark on this journey with us means more than words can express.

We wrote this book with the hope of making a positive impact on your life, and your dedication to reading it is a testament to your commitment to personal growth. We understand that embracing change and prioritizing your health can be a challenging endeavor, especially as we age, but your decision to explore the world of wall Pilates is a powerful step in the right direction.

As you dive into the exercises and principles laid out in these pages, we encourage you to be patient with yourself and trust in your own potential. Your well-being matters, and you deserve to live a life full of vitality and strength.

Thank you for entrusting us with your health and fitness journey. We are here to support and guide you every step of the way. Together, we can achieve remarkable transformations and celebrate the joy of better health.

With gratitude and warmest wishes,

Skylar Taylor.